MACROFUEL:

THE

MACRO DIET

COOKBOOK

FOR WOMEN

A woman's guide to balanced nutrition

2024

By Geneva J. Spoon

Copyright © 2023 by Geneva J. Spoon

All rights reserved. No part of this publication may be

reproduced, distributed, or transmitted in any form or by any

means, including photocopying, recording, or other electronic

or mechanical methods, without the prior written permission of

the publisher, except in the case of brief quotations embodied

in critical reviews and certain other non-commercial uses

permitted by copyright law.

Printed in the United States of America

Geneva J. Spoon

Contents

INTRODUCTION

Everyone wants to be healthy and that's understandable. However, sustaining health and wellbeing can frequently be a complex process for women in particular, necessitating a greater comprehension of dietary requirements. One strategy that has gained traction and shown to be quite helpful for women is the "Macro Diet," which involves keeping track of macronutrients. This book will examine the benefits of macronutrients for women's health, go over how to implement a macro diet, and offer crucial advice for macronutrient success.

The Power of Macros for Women's Health

Macronutrients, often referred to as "macros," are the essential nutrients the body needs in large quantities to function well. These macros include carbohydrates, proteins, and fats, and they play a pivotal role in the health and well-being of women.

1. Carbohydrates: Carbs are a primary source of energy. For women, ensuring an adequate intake of complex carbohydrates is crucial. They provide the energy needed for daily activities, support brain function, and maintain stable blood sugar levels. Fibre-rich carbs also aid digestion and promote satiety.

2. Proteins: Proteins are the building blocks of life. They are essential for tissue repair, muscle maintenance, and the production of hormones and enzymes. Women, in particular, can benefit from the muscle-preserving qualities of protein, which can support a healthy metabolism and maintain lean body mass.

3. Fats: Healthy fats, such as monounsaturated and polyunsaturated fats, are vital for hormone production, brain health, and absorption of fat-soluble vitamins. They also provide a feeling of fullness, which can aid in weight management.

Understanding the unique requirements for each macro is essential to employing them for women's health. It's crucial to keep in mind that several factors, such as age, activity level, and health objectives, influence the optimal macro balance. Women who follow a well-planned macro diet can enhance their athletic performance, manage health issues like PCOS or hormone imbalances, and maintain a healthy weight.

How to Follow a Macro Diet

Following a macro diet involves some measures in tracking and managing your daily intake of carbohydrates, proteins, and fats to ensure they align with your health goals. Here's how to get started:

1. **What are Your Goals?**

Clearly define your health and fitness objectives. Do you want to lose weight, gain muscle, or maintain your current weight? Your goals will dictate your macro ratios.

2. **Calculate Your Macros:** Use online calculators or consult with a nutritionist to determine your recommended daily macronutrient intake. This involves identifying your daily caloric needs and splitting those calories into the three macronutrient categories.

3. **Food Selection:** Choose high-quality sources of carbohydrates, proteins, and fats. For example, go for whole grains, lean meats, and healthy fats like avocados and nuts.

4. **Portion Control:** Measure your food portions to align with your macro goals. Food scales and measuring cups can be valuable tools in the early stages of your macro journey.

5. **Track Your Intake:** Utilize a food diary or mobile app to record your daily food consumption. This will help you monitor your macros and ensure they align with your goals.

6. **Adjust as Necessary:** Review your progress often, and if necessary, make changes to your macros. It's important to be flexible in your approach because your body's needs may alter over time.

Tips for Success with Macro Nutrition

1. Stay Consistent: Consistency is key. Make tracking your macros a daily habit.

2. Seek Professional Guidance: If you're new to macro tracking, consider consulting a registered dietician or nutritionist to ensure you're following a balanced and healthy diet.

3. Balance Micronutrients: While macros are essential, don't forget about micronutrients. Ensure you're getting a variety of vitamins and minerals through a diverse diet.

4. Listen to Your Body: Pay attention to hunger cues and adjust your macros based on your energy levels and satiety.

5. Be Patient: Results may not be immediate, and it's essential to be patient with your progress. Remember, slow and steady changes are often more sustainable.

There is no denying macros' beneficial effects on women's health. A macro diet that is well-planned can be an effective strategy for obtaining and preserving health and wellbeing. Women can maximize the health and wellness benefits of macronutrients by knowing the function of each one, adhering to a regimen, and paying attention to key advice. **Now let's get to the recipes!**

CHAPTER 1: BREAKFAST ENERGIZERS

- Protein-Packed Morning Meals:

1. **Veggie-Packed Omelette:**

   - Ingredients:

     - 2 large eggs

     - Chopped bell peppers, onions, and spinach

     - Diced tomatoes

     - Salt, pepper, and your choice of herbs

     - Olive oil for cooking

   - Instructions:

   1. Whisk the eggs and season with salt, pepper, and herbs.

   2. Heat a pan with a bit of olive oil and sauté the vegetables until tender.

   3. Pour the eggs over the veggies and cook until set. Fold the omelette in half and serve.

2. **Greek Yogurt Parfait:**

- Ingredients:

  - Greek yogurt

  - Fresh berries (e.g., strawberries, blueberries)

  - Honey or maple syrup

  - Granola

- Instructions:

  1. Layer Greek yogurt, berries, and granola in a glass or bowl.

  2. Drizzle with honey or maple syrup for added sweetness.

3. **Spinach and Feta Scramble:**

- Ingredients:

  - 2 large eggs

  - Chopped spinach

  - Crumbled feta cheese

- Diced tomatoes

- Salt, pepper, and olive oil

- Instructions:

1. Heat a pan with a bit of olive oil.

2. Whisk the eggs and season with salt and pepper.

3. Add chopped spinach and diced tomatoes to the pan and sauté until wilted.

4. Pour the whisked eggs over the vegetables, add crumbled feta, and scramble until fully cooked.

4. **Quinoa Breakfast Bowl:**

- Ingredients:

- Cooked quinoa

- Greek yogurt

- Sliced strawberries and bananas

- Almonds or walnuts

- Honey or maple syrup

- Instructions:

1. Place cooked quinoa in a bowl.

2. Top with Greek yogurt and sliced fruits.

3. Sprinkle with nuts and drizzle with honey or maple syrup for extra flavor.

5. Cottage Cheese Pancakes:

- Ingredients:

- 1 cup cottage cheese

- 2 large eggs

- 1/4 cup flour (e.g., whole wheat or almond flour)

- 1/2 teaspoon baking powder

- Vanilla extract (optional)

- Instructions:

1. Mix cottage cheese, eggs, flour, and baking powder (and vanilla, if using).

2. Heat a non-stick pan and cook small pancakes until golden on both sides.

6. Smoked Salmon and Avocado Toast:

- Ingredients:

  - 2 slices of whole grain bread

  - Smoked salmon slices

  - Sliced avocado

  - Red onion slices (optional)

  - Fresh dill and lemon juice

- Instructions:

1. Toast the bread slices.

2. Top with smoked salmon, sliced avocado, and red onion if desired.

3. Sprinkle with fresh dill and a squeeze of lemon juice.

7. High-Protein Vegan Smoothie:

- Ingredients:

  - 1 cup almond milk (or your choice of milk)

  - 1 scoop of plant-based protein powder

  - 1/2 cup silken tofu

  - Frozen berries or a ripe banana

  - A handful of spinach or kale

- Instructions:

1. Blend almond milk, protein powder, silken tofu, fruits, and greens until smooth.

2. Adjust sweetness with a bit of honey or maple syrup if desired.

These additional recipes offer a variety of options to kick-start your

day with a protein-packed morning meal. Enjoy your nutritious and

delicious breakfast!

Balanced Carbs to Start the Day:

1. **Oatmeal with Nut Butter:**

   - Ingredients:

     - 1/2 cup rolled oats

     - 1 cup almond milk (or your choice of milk)

     - 1 tablespoon nut butter (e.g., almond, peanut, or cashew)

     - Sliced bananas

     - Cinnamon and a drizzle of honey (optional)

- Instructions:

1. Cook oats in milk until they reach your desired consistency.

2. Top with nut butter, sliced bananas, a sprinkle of cinnamon, and a drizzle of honey if desired.

2. **Whole Grain Toast with Avocado:**

- Ingredients:

  - 2 slices of whole grain bread

  - 1 ripe avocado

  - Salt and pepper to taste

  - Sliced tomatoes or radishes (optional)

- Instructions:

1. Toast the bread slices.

2. Mash the ripe avocado and spread it on the toast.

3. Season with salt and pepper and add sliced tomatoes or radishes for extra flavor.

3. Quinoa Breakfast Burrito:

- Ingredients:

  - Cooked quinoa

  - Black beans

  - Salsa

  - Sliced avocado

  - Whole grain tortilla

- Instructions:

1. Warm the tortilla.

2. Layer cooked quinoa, black beans, salsa, and sliced avocado.

3. Roll into a burrito and enjoy.

4. **Sweet Potato and Chickpea Hash:**

- Ingredients:

  - Diced sweet potatoes

  - Cooked chickpeas

  - Red bell peppers

  - Diced onions

  - Olive oil, salt, and pepper

- Instructions:

1. Toss sweet potatoes, chickpeas, bell peppers, and onions in olive oil, salt, and pepper.

2. Roast in the oven until tender and slightly crispy.

3. Serve as a hearty hash.

5. **Multigrain Pancakes:**

- Ingredients:

  - 1 cup multigrain pancake mix

  - 1/2 cup milk (dairy or non-dairy)

  - Sliced bananas or blueberries

  - Maple syrup

- Instructions:

  1. Mix pancake mix with milk until you have a smooth batter.

  2. Cook pancakes on a griddle and top with sliced bananas or blueberries.

  3. Drizzle with maple syrup for sweetness.

These balanced carb recipes provide a mix of grains, legumes, and veggies to start your day with sustained energy and delicious flavors. Enjoy your wholesome breakfast!

Healthy Fats for Sustained Energy:

1. Chia Seed Pudding:

- Ingredients:

  - 2 tablespoons chia seeds

  - 1 cup almond milk (or your choice of milk)

  - 1/2 teaspoon vanilla extract

  - Fresh fruit (e.g., berries or sliced kiwi)

- Instructions:

1. Mix chia seeds, almond milk, and vanilla extract in a jar. Stir well.

2. Refrigerate overnight or for at least 2 hours until the mixture thickens.

3. Serve with fresh fruit on top.

2. **Nuts and Seeds Smoothie:**

   - Ingredients:

     - 1 cup almond milk (or your choice of milk)

     - 1/4 cup mixed nuts and seeds (e.g., almonds, walnuts, flaxseeds, chia seeds)

     - 1 ripe banana

     - A drizzle of honey (optional)

   - Instructions:

   1. Blend almond milk, nuts, seeds, and banana until smooth.

   2. Add honey if you prefer additional sweetness.

These recipes provide protein, balanced carbs, and healthy fats to start your day with energy and nutrition. You can adjust the nutrients to fit your taste. Enjoy your protein-packed, balanced breakfast!

Lean Proteins for Midday Fuel:

1. **Grilled Chicken Salad:**

  - Ingredients:

    - Grilled chicken breast

    - Mixed greens (e.g., lettuce, spinach)

    - Cherry tomatoes

    - Sliced cucumbers

    - Balsamic vinaigrette

  - Instructions:

  1. Slice the grilled chicken.

  2. Toss mixed greens, cherry tomatoes, and cucumbers in a

bowl.

3. Top with grilled chicken and drizzle with balsamic vinaigrette.

2. Salmon and Asparagus Foil Pack:

- Ingredients:

  - Salmon fillet

  - Fresh asparagus spears

  - Lemon slices

  - Olive oil, salt, and pepper

- Instructions:

1. Place the salmon fillet on a sheet of foil.

2. Arrange asparagus spears and lemon slices around the salmon.

3. Drizzle with olive oil, season with salt and pepper, and seal the foil into a packet.

4. Bake in the oven until salmon is cooked and asparagus is tender.

3. Turkey and Avocado Wrap:

- Ingredients:

  - Sliced turkey breast

  - Sliced avocado

  - Whole grain wrap

  - Baby spinach or arugula

  - Greek yogurt or hummus (as a spread)

- Instructions:

  1. Lay out a whole grain wrap.

  2. Spread Greek yogurt or hummus on the wrap.

  3. Layer sliced turkey, avocado, and fresh greens.

  4. Roll up the wrap and enjoy.

4. Tofu Stir-Fry:

- Ingredients:

  - Firm tofu, cubed

  - Mixed stir-fry vegetables (e.g., broccoli, bell peppers, carrots)

  - Soy sauce or teriyaki sauce

  - Ginger and garlic for flavor

- Instructions:

  1. Stir-fry tofu and mixed vegetables in a pan with a bit of oil.

  2. Season with soy sauce or teriyaki sauce, ginger, and garlic.

  3. Serve over brown rice or quinoa.

5. Lentil and Chickpea Salad:

- Ingredients:

  - Cooked lentils and chickpeas

  - Chopped cucumbers and tomatoes

  - Red onion, finely diced

- Fresh parsley

- Lemon vinaigrette

- Instructions:

1. Combine cooked lentils, chickpeas, cucumbers, tomatoes, red onion, and fresh parsley in a bowl.

2. Dress with lemon vinaigrette for added flavor.

Smart Carb Choices:

1. Quinoa and Black Bean Salad:

- Ingredients:

  - Cooked quinoa

  - Cooked black beans

  - Chopped bell peppers

  - Chopped red onions

- Lime juice and cilantro

- Instructions:

   1. Combine quinoa, black beans, bell peppers, and red onions.

   2. Squeeze fresh lime juice and add cilantro for flavor.

2. **Whole Wheat Pasta with Pesto:**

  - Ingredients:

    - Whole wheat pasta

    - Homemade or store-bought pesto sauce

    - Cherry tomatoes

    - Fresh basil leaves

  - Instructions:

   1. Cook whole wheat pasta until al dente.

   2. Toss with pesto sauce and top with halved cherry tomatoes and fresh basil leaves.

3. **Sweet Potato and Black Bean Burrito Bowl:**

   - Ingredients:

     - Roasted sweet potato cubes

     - Black beans

     - Cooked brown rice

     - Salsa and guacamole

     - Fresh cilantro

   - Instructions:

   1. Layer brown rice, black beans, roasted sweet potatoes, and salsa in a bowl.

   2. Top with guacamole and fresh cilantro.

4. **Whole Grain Breakfast Burrito:**

   - Ingredients:

     - Scrambled eggs or tofu (for a vegan option)

- Whole grain tortilla

- Sliced avocado

- Salsa and black beans

- Spinach or kale

- Instructions:

1. Place scrambled eggs or tofu on a whole grain tortilla.

2. Add sliced avocado, salsa, black beans, and greens.

3. Roll into a burrito and enjoy.

5. **Mushroom and Spinach Stuffed Bell Peppers:**

- Ingredients:

- Bell peppers

- Quinoa or brown rice

- Sautéed mushrooms and spinach

- Marinara sauce

- Grated mozzarella cheese (optional)

- Instructions:

1. Cut the tops off bell peppers and remove seeds.

2. Stuff with a mixture of quinoa or brown rice, sautéed mushrooms, and spinach.

3. Top with marinara sauce and bake until peppers are tender.

4. Optionally, sprinkle with grated mozzarella before serving.

Nutrient-Dense Veggie Sides:

1. **Roasted Brussels Sprouts:**

- Ingredients:

- Brussels sprouts, trimmed and halved

- Olive oil, salt, and pepper

- Grated Parmesan cheese (optional)

- Instructions:

1. Toss Brussels sprouts in olive oil, salt, and pepper.

2. Roast in the oven until tender and slightly crispy.

3. Sprinkle with grated Parmesan cheese if desired.

2. Garlic Sautéed Spinach:

- Ingredients:

  - Fresh baby spinach

  - Minced garlic

  - Olive oil, salt, and pepper

- Instructions:

1. Heat olive oil in a pan and sauté minced garlic until fragrant.

2. Add fresh spinach and cook until wilted.

3. Season with salt and pepper.

3. **Garlic Roasted Broccoli:**

- Ingredients:

  - Fresh broccoli florets

  - Minced garlic

  - Olive oil, salt, and pepper

- Instructions:

  1. Toss broccoli with minced garlic, olive oil, salt, and pepper.

  2. Roast in the oven until crisp-tender and slightly browned.

4. **Mashed Cauliflower with Chives:**

- Ingredients:

  - Cooked cauliflower florets

  - Chopped chives

  - Greek yogurt or sour cream

  - Salt and pepper

- Instructions:

1. Mash cooked cauliflower with chopped chives, Greek yogurt or sour cream, salt, and pepper.

2. Serve as a healthier alternative to mashed potatoes.

5. Cucumber and Tomato Salad:

- Ingredients:

  - Sliced cucumbers and tomatoes

  - Red onion, thinly sliced

  - Fresh basil or mint leaves

  - Olive oil and balsamic vinegar

  - Salt and pepper

- Instructions:

1. Combine sliced cucumbers, tomatoes, red onion, and fresh herbs in a bowl.

2. Drizzle with olive oil and balsamic vinegar.

3. Season with salt and pepper and toss to combine.

Complete Proteins for Dinner:

1. Baked Lemon Herb Salmon:

- Ingredients:

  - Salmon fillets

  - Fresh lemon juice

  - Chopped fresh herbs (e.g., dill, parsley)

  - Minced garlic

- Instructions:

1. Marinate salmon fillets with lemon juice, herbs, and minced garlic.

2. Bake in the oven until the salmon is flaky and cooked through.

2. Grilled Tofu and Vegetable Skewers:

- Ingredients:

  - Cubed firm tofu

  - Bell peppers, zucchini, and red onion chunks

  - Marinade (olive oil, soy sauce, garlic, and spices)

- Instructions:

  1. Thread tofu and vegetable chunks onto skewers.

  2. Brush with the marinade and grill until veggies are tender and tofu is lightly browned.

3. Lentil and Quinoa Stuffed Bell Peppers:

- Ingredients:

  - Bell peppers

  - Cooked lentils and quinoa

  - Chopped tomatoes, onions, and herbs

- Spices and vegetable broth

- Instructions:

1. Cut the tops off bell peppers and remove seeds.

2. Stuff with a mixture of cooked lentils, quinoa, chopped tomatoes, onions, herbs, and spices.

3. Bake until peppers are tender.

4. **Chicken and Vegetable Stir-Fry:**

- Ingredients:

- Sliced chicken breast

- Mixed stir-fry vegetables

- Stir-fry sauce (soy sauce, ginger, garlic)

- Instructions:

1. Stir-fry sliced chicken in a pan.

2. Add mixed vegetables and stir-fry sauce.

3. Cook until chicken is cooked through and veggies are tender.

5. Shrimp and Avocado Salad:

- Ingredients:

  - Cooked shrimp

  - Sliced avocado

  - Mixed greens

  - Cilantro and lime dressing

- Instructions:

1. Combine cooked shrimp, sliced avocado, mixed greens, and cilantro.

2. Drizzle with lime dressing for flavor.

Healthy Carbs and Fiber:

1. Spaghetti Squash with Tomato and Basil:

- Ingredients:

  - Roasted spaghetti squash

  - Fresh tomato and basil sauce

  - Grated Parmesan cheese (optional)

- Instructions:

  1. Roast spaghetti squash and scrape out the strands.

  2. Top with a fresh tomato and basil sauce.

  3. Sprinkle with grated Parmesan cheese if desired.

2. Chickpea and Spinach Curry:

- Ingredients:

  - Chickpeas

- Fresh spinach

- Curry sauce (tomato, spices, coconut milk)

- Instructions:

1. Combine chickpeas, fresh spinach, and curry sauce in a pot.

2. Simmer until the spinach wilts and the flavors meld.

3. **Whole Wheat Pasta Primavera:**

- Ingredients:

- Whole wheat pasta

- Sautéed mixed vegetables (e.g., bell peppers, broccoli, cherry tomatoes)

- Olive oil and garlic

- Instructions:

1. Cook whole wheat pasta until al dente.

2. Toss with sautéed mixed vegetables, olive oil, and garlic.

4. Brown Rice and Black Bean Bowl:

- Ingredients:

  - Cooked brown rice

  - Black beans

  - Sliced avocado

  - Salsa and lime juice

- Instructions:

1. Layer brown rice, black beans, sliced avocado, and salsa in a bowl.

2. Drizzle with lime juice for added flavor.

5. Baked Sweet Potato Fries:

- Ingredients:

- Sliced sweet potatoes

- Olive oil, paprika, and salt

- Instructions:

1. Toss sweet potato slices in olive oil, paprika, and salt.

2. Bake in the oven until they are crispy and browned.

Filling, Nutrient-Rich Sides:

1. **Quinoa and Vegetable Salad:**

   - Ingredients:

   - Cooked quinoa

   - Roasted or grilled vegetables (e.g., bell peppers, zucchini, asparagus)

   - Fresh herbs and vinaigrette dressing

   - Instructions:

1. Combine cooked quinoa and roasted or grilled vegetables.

2. Add fresh herbs and dress with vinaigrette for added flavor.

2. **Steamed Broccoli with Garlic Butter:**

- Ingredients:

  - Fresh broccoli florets

  - Minced garlic

  - Melted butter (or a butter alternative)

- Instructions:

  1. Steam broccoli until tender-crisp.

  2. Toss with minced garlic and melted butter.

Protein-Packed Snacks:

1. Greek Yogurt Parfait:

- Ingredients:

  - Greek yogurt

  - Fresh berries (e.g., strawberries, blueberries)

  - Honey or maple syrup

  - Granola

- Instructions:

  1. Layer Greek yogurt, berries, and granola in a glass or bowl.

  2. Drizzle with honey or maple syrup for added sweetness.

2. Hard-Boiled Eggs with Hummus:

- Ingredients:

  - Hard-boiled eggs

  - Hummus for dipping

- Instructions:

  1. Slice hard-boiled eggs in half.

  2. Serve with hummus for a protein-packed snack.

3. Protein-Packed Energy Bites

- Ingredients:

  - Rolled oats

  - Peanut butter or almond butter

  - Honey

  - Chia seeds

  - Protein powder

- Instructions:

1. Mix rolled oats, nut butter, honey, chia seeds, and protein powder in a bowl.

2. Roll into small bites and refrigerate until firm.

Smart Carb Snacking:

1. **Apple Slices with Almond Butter:**

- Ingredients:

  - Apple slices

  - Almond butter

- Instructions:

1. Slice apples.

2. Dip in almond butter for a satisfying snack.

2. **Whole Wheat Crackers with Tuna Salad:**

- Ingredients:

  - Whole wheat crackers

  - Tuna salad (canned tuna, Greek yogurt, mustard, chopped pickles, and spices)

- Instructions:

  1. Top whole wheat crackers with tuna salad for a tasty snack.

3. **Veggie Sticks with Hummus:**

- Ingredients:

  - Carrot, celery, and cucumber sticks

  - Hummus for dipping

- Instructions:

  1. Slice veggies into sticks.

2. Dip in hummus for a nutritious snack.

Healthy Fats on the Go:

1. **Avocado Toast on Whole Grain Bread:**

   - Ingredients:

     - Whole grain toast

     - Mashed avocado

     - Sliced tomatoes

     - Sprinkle of sea salt and black pepper

   - Instructions:

     1. Spread mashed avocado on whole grain toast.

     2. Top with sliced tomatoes and a sprinkle of sea salt and black

pepper.

2. **Trail Mix:**

- Ingredients:

  - Mixed nuts (e.g., almonds, walnuts)

  - Dried fruits (e.g., raisins, apricots)

  - Dark chocolate chips

- Instructions:

1. Mix nuts, dried fruits, and dark chocolate chips in a portable container for an on-the-go snack.

3. **Chia Pudding with Berries:**

- Ingredients:

  - Chia seeds

- Almond milk

- Fresh berries

- Drizzle of honey (optional)

- Instructions:

1. Combine chia seeds and almond milk in a jar.

2. Refrigerate until the mixture thickens.

3. Top with fresh berries and drizzle with honey if desired.

CHAPTER 5: SWEET AND SATISFYING DESSERTS

-Low-Guilt Sweet Treats:

1. **Frozen Banana Bites:**

   - Ingredients:

     - Sliced bananas

     - Almond or peanut butter

     - Dark chocolate chips

   - Instructions:

     1. Spread a small amount of nut butter on banana slices.

     2. Sandwich them together and dip in melted dark chocolate.

     3. Place on a tray and freeze until chocolate hardens.

2. **Yogurt Parfait with Berries and Honey:**

   - Ingredients:

     - Greek yogurt

- Fresh berries (e.g., strawberries, blueberries)

- Drizzle of honey

- Instructions:

1. Layer Greek yogurt, fresh berries, and a drizzle of honey in a glass.

2. Repeat for a delicious parfait.

3. Dark Chocolate-Dipped Strawberries:

- Ingredients:

- Fresh strawberries

- Dark chocolate (70% cocoa or higher)

- Instructions:

1. Melt dark chocolate in a microwave or on a stovetop.

2. Dip strawberries in melted chocolate and place on a tray.

3. Let them cool until the chocolate hardens.

Healthy Dessert Substitutions:

1. Avocado Chocolate Mousse:

- Ingredients:

  - Ripe avocados

  - Unsweetened cocoa powder

  - Maple syrup or honey

  - Vanilla extract

- Instructions:

1. Blend avocados, cocoa powder, sweetener, and vanilla extract until smooth.

2. Chill in the refrigerator before serving.

2. Baked Apples with Cinnamon and Nuts:

- Ingredients:

  - Apples, cored and sliced

  - Cinnamon

  - Chopped nuts (e.g., almonds or walnuts)

- Instructions:

  1. Sprinkle apple slices with cinnamon and chopped nuts.

  2. Bake in the oven until apples are tender.

3. Chia Seed Pudding with Fresh Fruit:

- Ingredients:

  - Chia seeds

  - Almond milk (or your choice of milk)

  - Fresh fruit (e.g., sliced mango, kiwi)

  - Drizzle of agave nectar

- Instructions:

1. Mix chia seeds and almond milk in a jar.

2. Refrigerate until the mixture thickens.

3. Top with fresh fruit and a drizzle of agave nectar.

Desserts to Satisfy Your Sweet Tooth:

1. **Homemade Berry Sorbet:**

   - Ingredients:

     - Frozen mixed berries

     - Greek yogurt

     - Honey

   - Instructions:

     1. Blend frozen berries, Greek yogurt, and honey until smooth.

     2. Freeze for a couple of hours before serving.

2. **Oatmeal Raisin Cookies:**

- Ingredients:

  - Rolled oats

  - Raisins

  - Cinnamon and nutmeg

  - Maple syrup

- Instructions:

1. Mix rolled oats, raisins, cinnamon, nutmeg, and maple syrup in a bowl.

2. Form into cookies and bake until golden brown.

3. **Fruit Salad with Mint and Lime:**

- Ingredients:

- Fresh fruit (e.g., watermelon, pineapple, berries)

- Chopped fresh mint

- Lime juice and zest

- Drizzle of honey (optional)

- Instructions:

1. Combine fresh fruit, chopped mint, lime juice, and zest in a

bowl.

2. Drizzle with honey if desired.

For women of all ages, maintaining good health is of utmost importance. Nutrition is a major factor in women's health, and obtaining general well-being requires a grasp of macronutrients, or "macros. Let us explore the ways that macros can improve women's energy and vitality, help with weight management, and affect hormone balance

Macros and Hormonal Balance:

Hormonal fluctuations are a natural part of a woman's life, from puberty to menopause. Nutrition can play a significant role in balancing these hormones, leading to better overall health.

Proteins: Adequate protein intake supports the production of essential hormones. Amino acids from protein sources are building blocks for hormones like insulin and growth hormones. Lean proteins, such as poultry, fish, and tofu, can promote hormonal stability.

Fats: The production of progesterone and estrogen, two sex hormones, depends on healthy fats. Including foods like almonds, avocados, and olive oil can support the preservation of hormonal balance. Women suffering from PMS or menopausal symptoms can benefit from the anti-inflammatory qualities of omega-3 fatty acids, which are found in fatty seafood like salmon.

Carbohydrates: In addition to providing fiber, complex carbs from fruits, vegetables, and whole grains also help to maintain stable blood sugar levels. This is especially important for women who have diabetes or PCOS because blood sugar swings can throw off the hormonal balance.

Macros and Weight Management:

Weight management is a common concern among women. Macronutrients can be strategically utilized to maintain a healthy weight.

Proteins: A high-protein diet can help women feel full and reduce overall calorie intake. It also supports muscle maintenance, aiding in fat loss. Protein-rich foods provide a thermic effect, meaning your body burns more calories during digestion.

Fats: Healthy fats promote satiety and can reduce cravings for unhealthy, calorie-dense foods. These fats also support hormone regulation, which is key to weight management.

Carbohydrates: Balanced carbohydrate consumption is essential. While low-carb diets can be effective for some, complex carbohydrates are necessary for sustained energy, especially for active women. Balancing carb intake can help prevent energy dips and overeating.

Macros for Energy and Vitality:

Maintaining energy levels and vitality is essential for women, who often juggle busy schedules, careers, and family responsibilities.

Proteins: Protein provides steady, long-lasting energy. Incorporating it into meals and snacks can help avoid energy crashes. Additionally, protein supports muscle health, which is important for daily activities and overall vitality.

Fats: Healthy fats, like those found in nuts and seeds, provide a concentrated source of energy. These fats are also essential for brain health and cognitive function, which is vital for women in various roles.

Carbohydrates: Carbohydrates are the body's primary energy source. Whole grains, fruits, and vegetables provide essential nutrients and fiber that keep energy levels stable. The key is to choose complex carbs, which are slowly digested, preventing blood sugar spikes and crashes.

It is critical for women's health to comprehend macronutrients and how they affect energy levels, weight management, and hormonal balance. Achieving the ideal ratios of fats, proteins, and carbs can enable women to live longer, healthier lives. To ensure that every woman has the best possible health, keep in mind that speaking with a healthcare professional or nutritionist can assist customize macronutrient consumption to meet her needs and goals.

CONCLUSION

Mastering Macros: Tips for Macro Meal Prep, Creating Balanced Macro Meal Plans, and Stocking Your Macro Diet Pantry

The macro diet, which focuses on the balance of macronutrients—proteins, fats, and carbohydrates—has gained popularity for its ability to promote overall health, help with weight management, and boost energy. To make the most of your macro diet, consider these essential tips for macro meal prep, creating well-balanced macro meal plans, and stocking your pantry with the right ingredients.

Tips for Macro Meal Prep:

1. Establish Your Objectives: Establish your objectives, whether they be to maintain a healthy diet, increase muscle, or lose weight. As a result, your macronutrient ratios will change.

2. Determine Your Macros: - Determine your daily macro requirements by taking into account your age, gender, activity level, and goals. This is where a number of online calculators come in handy.

3. Create a Meal Plan: - Create a meal plan that complements your macro objectives. Maintain the proper ratios of carbohydrates, lipids, and proteins at every meal.

4. Batch Cooking:

  - Prepare larger quantities of your favorite macro-friendly dishes and portion them into containers for easy access throughout the week.

5. Use a Food Scale:

  - Invest in a kitchen scale to measure and portion your foods accurately. This ensures you stick to your macro goals.

Creating Balanced Macro Meal Plans:

1. Focus on Lean Proteins:

  - Include lean protein sources like chicken, turkey, fish, tofu, and legumes in your meal plans. Protein helps maintain muscle and provides a feeling of fullness.

2. Choose Healthy Fats:

- Incorporate sources of healthy fats such as avocados, nuts, seeds, and olive oil. Healthy fats are vital for hormone production and overall well-being.

3. Opt for Complex Carbs:

- Prioritize complex carbohydrates like whole grains, sweet potatoes, and fruits. They release energy gradually, preventing blood sugar spikes.

4. Experiment with Recipes:

- Keep your meal plan exciting by exploring new recipes that adhere to your macro goals. Online resources and cookbooks offer a wealth of inspiration.

5. Monitor Portion Sizes:

   - Be mindful of portion sizes to avoid overeating and stay within your macro limits. Smaller, well-balanced meals can keep you on track.

Macro Diet Pantry Essentials:

1. Whole Grains:

   - Stock up on whole grains like brown rice, quinoa, oats, and whole wheat pasta to ensure a steady supply of complex carbs.

2. Lean Proteins:

   - Have lean protein sources readily available, such as canned tuna, chicken breast, tofu, and beans.

3. Healthy Fats:

  - Keep a variety of healthy fats in your pantry, including extra virgin olive oil, avocados, and a selection of nuts and seeds.

4. Canned and Frozen Vegetables:

  - To ensure you always have a source of veggies, keep canned and frozen options like spinach, peas, and green beans on hand.

5. Condiments and Spices:

  - Flavor your meals with condiments and spices like mustard, low-sodium soy sauce, herbs, and spices. They can enhance the taste of your macro-friendly dishes.

6. Low-Sugar Snacks:

  - Opt for low-sugar snack options such as rice cakes, nut butter, and unsweetened yogurt for between-meal satisfaction.

You can achieve your dietary goals while enjoying delicious and satisfying meals with careful macro meal preparation, well-planned meal plans, and a pantry stocked with the essentials. Whether you're working towards weight management, muscle gain, or simply a healthier lifestyle, the macro diet is a versatile approach to achieving your health and nutrition goals.

www.ingramcontent.com/pod-product-compliance
Lightning Source LLC
Chambersburg PA
CBHW050849260726
48660CB00006B/2534